In the pursuit of technological progress, we have become very much engrossed in the material world and have begun to forget the spiritual world. In the cycle of everyday life, making money has become our priority, and time has become the vassal of money. Sometimes we take a quick glance at the sky, which has grown distant from us and is not as lovely as it was in our carefree childhood. We invented computers and rockets, but we know absolutely nothing about ourselves.

We don't know why our hearts beat and what we live for, what thought is and what the meaning of life is. We have gradually begun to forget about the method of healing, which was used by mankind in ancient times, when there were no medicines and medical equipment. Of course, many books have been written on this subject, but the high pace of life and lack of time does not allow many people to study all these disparate works. The purpose of this book is to simplify the acquisition of this knowledge by the average person and to try to place in his mind an idea which he can later develop with more knowledge. The reader is offered a brief reference book on the treatment of people by the biological field.

Copyright © 2023 Victor Grigorev.
Library of Congress registration number TXu 2-404-631

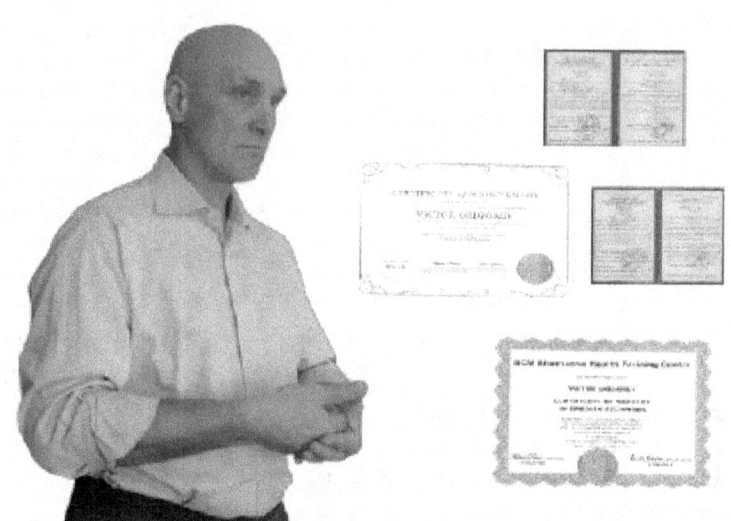

Victor Grigoriev's career began in the distant 1991, when he was trained in the Russian international center of experimental parapsychology "Black Lotus Temple of Immortality" and received the highest qualification of an instructor in diagnostics and biofield correction. In 2008, he successfully passed the exams in classical massage at the Moscow Institute of Restorative Medicine. In 2014, he was certified by the Alternative Health Training Center in the USA. Thirty years of experience practicing in this service area prompted him to write a book on the unconventional treatment method.

Victor Grigorev

BIOFIELD

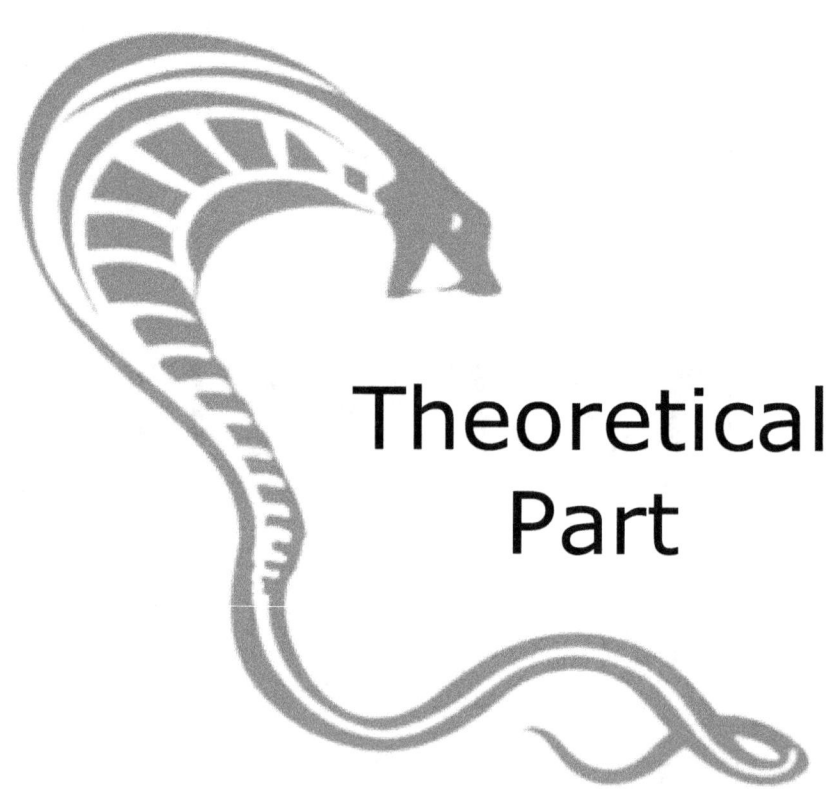

Theoretical Part

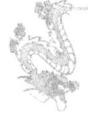 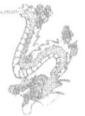

All of the following is concise but sufficient to understand the essence of the information obtained from available information sources and is only a practical guide for those who want to try to develop in themselves the abilities laid down by nature to diagnose and treat various diseases. This will improve your health and broaden your level of worldview. This book contains the basic provisions of treatment of the biological field (aura, biofield) of a person by correcting it by applying hands and mental passes in order to heal from many diseases. Only those who overcome the inner barrier of distrust in their abilities can master these abilities.

The doctrine of practical application of biological energy was first developed by yogis of ancient India. Jesus Christ also treated people with the power of thought and this fact is recorded in the Bible.

4

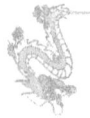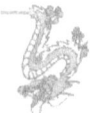

In medieval Europe healers were mercilessly executed by the Holy Inquisition to fight heresy. In Brazil Joao Teixeeira de Faria helped thousands of sick people from different countries. In Canada, Adam Dreamheeler healed people over long distances using photographs. In the Soviet Union, the healer Dzhuna was famous. This list can go on for a long time. The world community learned about the secrets of the human biofield after the publication of the books "Hypnotism" by Hiram Jackson, "Healing Magnetism" by Van-Ness Stilman, "Occult Treatment of Yogis" by Yogi Ramacharaka. Human beings get the necessary energy for the body to function in the right amount through food, water and space. The energy received from outside or generated in the body is distributed to all cells and organs and transformed into a biofield around the person. The process is reversible, i.e. the biofield can be transformed back into energy, by analogy with any other energy.

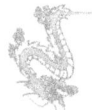 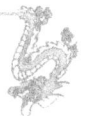

In the question of creation of the human being and his possibilities now much remains a mystery, but it is already clear that for work of an organism it is necessary not only receipt of chemical elements and organic compounds, but also receipt of energy from space. Yogi Prahlad Jani from India could do without water and food for a long time. Buddhist lama from Russia Dashi-Dorjo Itigelova died almost 100 years ago, but his body does not decompose and consumes energy from space until now.

The human spine has different polarities on opposite sides, and along it there are seven energy centers (chakras), which unite energy flows. They have their frequencies of oscillation in ascending order and their colors from red to purple, some people even see these colors. At the base of the spine is located the first chakra, which has a red color and the lowest frequency of vibration - this is the level of physical strength, the sexual chakra.

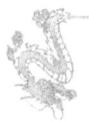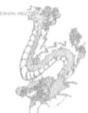

At the birth of a person
this center is developed more than others,
and the weakest is the opposite spiritual
chakra in the parietal zone, which has a
purple color and the highest frequency of
vibration. With time, this chakra develops
more strongly, but the sex chakra fades away.
This is why it is easier to stir up rage than
kindness in a young person, and the opposite
is true in old age. By applying red lighting and
rhythmic low-frequency music, one can
achieve good results in reanimating the work
of the sex chakra. For the development of the
spiritual chakra, blue light and high-frequency
meditation music are used. Green light is used
to treat the chakra that is located in the
middle of the spinal column and is green in
color. When one looks at the beauty of green
nature, one's heart is soothed.

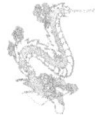
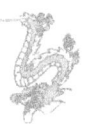

Energy centers

control the functioning of their specific organs. The red chakra is located in the perineum area and controls the sexual organs. Orange - opposite the pubis (intestines). Yellow - near the navel (liver and stomach). Green - on the chest (heart and lungs). Light blue - near the neck (throat and nose). Blue - in the center of the forehead (eyes). Purple - on the top of the head (brain). When all chakras work harmoniously, a person feels great and the biofield around him has the form of a large smooth cocoon of egg-shape. In case of diseases the cocoon is uneven. In a perfectly healthy person the biofield is felt at a distance of one or two elbows from the body, in a sick person - half an elbow or less. Before the death of a person, the biofield concentrates around the head and quickly disappears, while the weight decreases by several milligrams. The shape and size of the biofield is determined by the vine, frames, pendulum and hands.

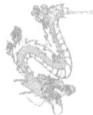
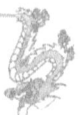

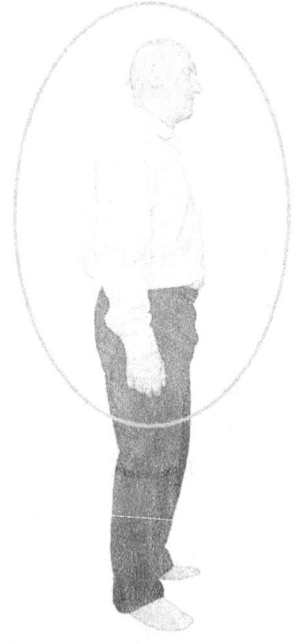
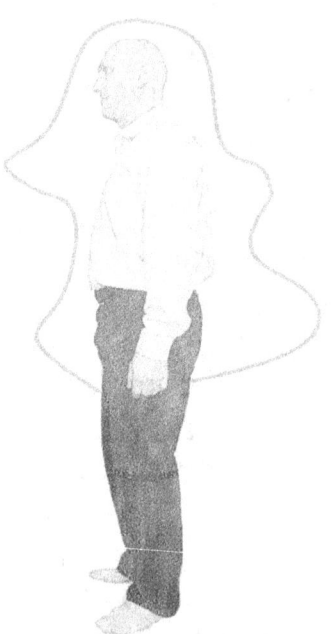

The man is healthy   The sick man

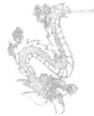 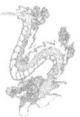

Nature has endowed man with hands with which he feels, touches, evaluates and helps the body in case of illness. When something hurts, we automatically put our hands on these places. Energy flows through our hands, which we transfer to the sore places. With our hands we can touch the biofield and make its correction in case of illnesses. Hands are a counter of information, and the vine and frames are only additional aids, with the help of which people still find underground water sources and mineral deposits. A person simply mentally tunes in to receive certain information and then receives it. By bringing the hands close to the patient's biofield, tingling, warmth, cold or resistance sensations may occur.

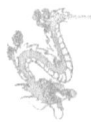 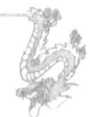

Energy flows
of all chakras are united. All components of the body are inextricably linked and separately their normal work is impossible. A diseased chakra is helped by other chakras, because the whole organism is interconnected and a person can heal himself by uncontrolled transfer of energy from another chakra only under the control of his subconscious mind. The second variant of treatment is the help of a healer who is able to align the patient's biofield by the power of thought and hands, as Indian yogis do. The aligned biofield accumulates energy in the affected organs and the person recovers. Through holes in the biofield speak about cancerous diseases, which are practically impossible to cure with hands, but with hands they can be diagnosed and treatment according to the scheme of traditional medicine can be prescribed in time. Detection of cancers in the early stage of the disease is the main problem in oncology today.

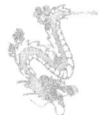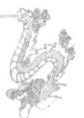

To provide quality help, a healer must be absolutely healthy and be able to quickly replenish his personal energy, and there are special exercises for this purpose. One must learn to relax deeply, concentrate attention and develop spatial imagination. The treatment should not be started without an emotional attitude, if you feel unwell and if you are unsure of your strength. Irritation leads to loss of energy. Self-confidence should not come from ignorance, but from a full understanding of the process. You need to work out your tactics and intuitively create your own treatment option for yourself, according to your skills and capabilities. Know that biofield correction is not enough for complete healing. It is necessary to expand the spiritual world of the patient, only then the success will be fixed for a long time.

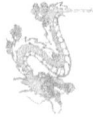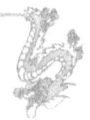

If possible,

you should familiarize yourself with the teachings of yoga and European literature on biological energy. You will definitely see the same thoughts from ancient teachings and modern interpretations on this issue. Later you will begin to realize about huge opportunities in case of mastering the knowledge of biological energy management, but you should never use them to the detriment of other people. You should never answer a person with rudeness for rudeness, take a pause in a conflict situation and it will go away. Be in nature more often, contemplate it with wonder and respect as if you were a guest on this planet. Love others as yourself, be kind to them and help them freely. When the mind is pure in thoughts, then the inner energy only increases. The practical part consists of 7 parts. Remember that you can start each subsequent part only after a good mastery of the previous part.

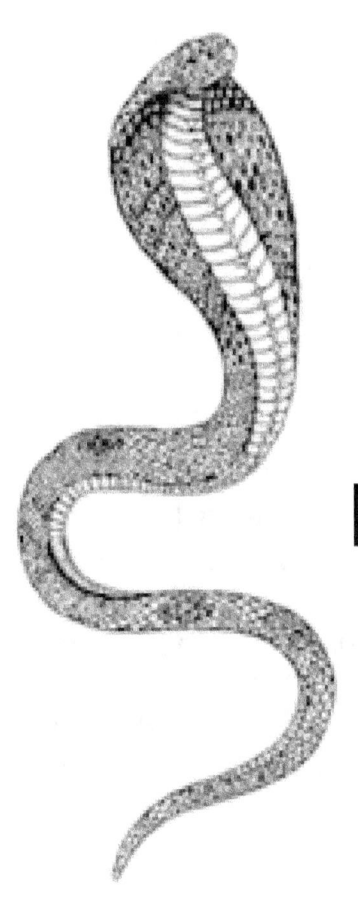

Practical Part

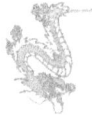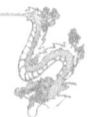

Relaxation

Relaxation is muscle and emotional relaxation. Calmness and   self-control help to gain energy and regain strength. Nature has   endowed us with the gift of deep relaxation since childhood, but with age this ability goes away. Constant subconscious muscle tension causes loss of energy and fatigue, so you need to learn deep relaxation and be able to focus on different muscles of the body.

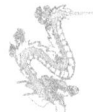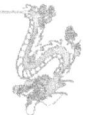

1. As you exhale, relax the muscles of your face and neck, and hang your head on your chest. Rotate your torso, with the hanging head also rotating easily.

2. With relaxed arms hanging loosely, make a few sweeps of the hands to the sides.

3. Sit on a chair and relax your back muscles, with your body tilted slightly forward.

4. While lying down, stretch and roll over.

5. Lying on your back close your eyes and relax on the exhalation, while holding your breath, check the relaxation of all parts of the body from the face to the feet. Pay special attention to the muscles of the face, eyes and mouth. As you inhale, tense the muscles and repeat the cycle again.

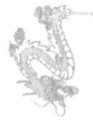 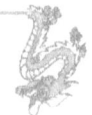

Concentration

Holding information about an object in short-term memory is called concentration of attention. We often involuntarily do this in our daily lives, staring thoughtfully at something for a few seconds. When the mind is focused on any point, all senses disappear and the surrounding world is not perceived. Use any time in transportation, at work and at home in a sitting or lying position to practice. The best time to practice is early morning or evening. You should achieve a steady result. Gradually increase your concentration time from a minute to 30 minutes.

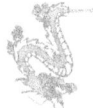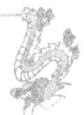

1. Sit on a chair, relax, breathe calmly, straighten your back, cross your legs, place your hands on your knees. Close your eyes and focus your attention on the monotonous sound of a hair dryer or rain, for example. Open your eyes and focus on any small object like a dot, a pencil or a book. Try not to blink. Examine the pencil carefully and find the smallest details in it. Your attention may drift to another sound or object, this is a normal reaction. Do not resist what is happening, watch the thought go away and then gently return it to its place.

2. lying or sitting down, close your eyes and concentrate on the tip of your nose, your thoughts slowly calming down. When good results are achieved, you may see light.

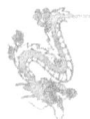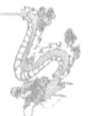

Spatial Imagination

After developing in yourself the concentration of attention, you can move on to exercises to develop spatial imagination, that is, learn to mentally model and determine the relationship between the individual elements of the image, change their mutual location and see them with inner vision in color and detail.

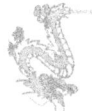 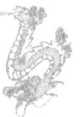

1. Look carefully at some object. Close your eyes and mentally imagine it in color and the smallest details, then open your eyes and compare it with the original. Repeat this exercise several times. After getting a good result, gradually move on to more difficult subjects, like art paintings.

2. Look at one object for a few minutes, then another. Close your eyes and mentally place one object on another, for example: a pen on a book.

3. Lying on your back, close your eyes and concentrate on your forehead. Visualize and hold in your mind for a few minutes very green grass, very white clouds, a very yellow yolk and a very blue sky.

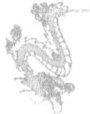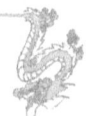

4. Close your eyes. Concentrate on the tip of your tongue and imagine the taste of a very sour lemon, then the taste of very sweet honey.

5. Mentally hold a jar of very hot water in the palms of your hands, then take very cold ice from the freezer.

6. Imagine a clear blue sky with slowly floating white clouds.

7. Open your eyes. Look at an artistic painting of nature. Imagine that you have entered it and are a participant in the events. Hear the birds chirping, smell the beautiful multicolored flowers and the movement of a warm gentle breeze.

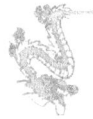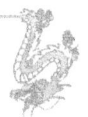

Energy intake through food

It is important to realize that our diet should be nutritious and varied. You should drink water at least 2 liters a day. It is desirable not to eat meat at all, especially fatty meat. Full-fledged protein can be obtained from leguminous plants, because the human body is closer to herbivores than to carnivores. Unlike animals, we have a long intestine, because it takes a long time to digest proteins from plant foods. The following is an example of a diet, but it should be adopted gradually in order to adapt the body to the new conditions.

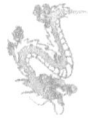 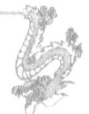

6:30 Dried apricots or prunes. Water-soaked buckwheat, wheat, oats or oat flakes. A glass of hot water with a spoonful of honey. Any non-acidic fruit. This breakfast cleanses the body of toxins.

11:30 Vegetables, fruits, fish, poultry, eggs, dairy products, coarse bread.

15:00 You can eat everything except fatty meat.

19:00 Vegetarian dinner no later than 4 hours before bedtime.

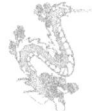
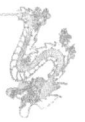

Recruitment of energy from the space around us

To master the technique of recruiting energy from the space around us, we need to learn rhythmic breathing. Normal work of lungs is necessary, so they should be developed. There may be difficulties in exhalation, but you need to overcome them. Do not hurry and do not forget to create a mental image of the flow of energy, breathe with the abdominal cavity. By the end of the second week of training there should be a feeling of increased vital energy, and after the final mastering of the technique fatigue and illness will lose power over the body. Exercise sitting or lying down 3 times a day for 10 minutes at any time before meals, but not late at night. It is desirable to perform the exercises in the presence of other people. Before each exercise, relax the muscles of the body well. Then follow these steps:

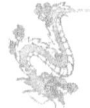
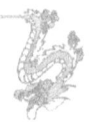

1. In the first week of exercise, take a slow deep breath for 8 seconds, then hold your breath for 8 seconds and exhale slowly for 8 seconds.

2. In the second week, close the right nostril with your finger and take a deep breath for 10 seconds, then hold your breath for 10 seconds and exhale for 10 seconds through the left nostril. After 10 cycles change the nostril.

3. In the third week, close the right nostril with your finger and take a deep breath for 15 seconds, then hold your breath for 10 seconds and exhale for 15 seconds through the left nostril. After 8 cycles change the nostril.

4. In the fourth week, close the right nostril with your finger and take a deep breath for 20 seconds, then hold your breath for 10 seconds and exhale for 20 seconds through the left nostril. After 6 cycles change the nostril.

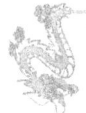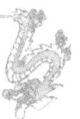

5. In the fifth week, do 3 sessions a day for 25 minutes. Close the right nostril with your finger and inhale deeply for 26 seconds, then hold your breath for 8 seconds and exhale for 26 seconds through the left nostril. After 5 cycles change the nostril.

The following is a procedure that is good for strengthening the cardiovascular system and enhancing the biofield.

6. Take a contrast shower twice a day for 4 minutes, starting with cold water and ending with hot water. Feel a surge of energy. Within 3 months, gradually increase the contrast of water to the maximum and increase the exercise time to 8 minutes.

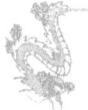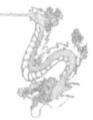

Gymnastics with rhythmic tension and relaxation will help to achieve great results in energy intake and distribution of energy throughout the body, but is not recommended for the elderly. Do the exercises below standing, feet shoulder width apart, arms hanging loosely, all muscles relaxed. Perform each exercise 4 times a day with a good flexion of the body. Inhale with a blow of air on the nasopharynx and short, which is why little air will enter the lungs. After the muscles are tensed, energy deficit will be formed in the body and it will start coming through the skin. Through the mouth make a sharp noisy exhalation with the whole chest, after that relax and further:

7. Inhale, throw your relaxed arms to the sides and bring them behind your back by inertia, bend your torso backwards, throw back your head, tense up, clench your fists and hold your breath for 4 seconds. Then exhale, bend your torso forward and relax completely, hands almost touching the floor. Hold this pose for 4 seconds.

27

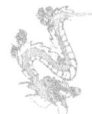
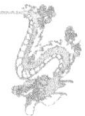

8. Inhale, lock your hands and bring them to the right side behind your head, improvising a swing of an axe. At the same time, bend your body backwards, tilt your head, tense up and hold your breath for 4 seconds. Next, exhale, relax, lower your arms in a circle on the left side, bend your torso forward, unclasp your hands and hang them loosely. Stay in this pose for 4 seconds. Then make swings of the axe from different sides.

9. Inhale, quickly turn the relaxed body counterclockwise and at the same time throw the right arm forward at the forehead level by inertia, and take the left arm backwards. The head turns together with the torso. At the end of the trajectory tense up, clench your fists, hold your breath for 4 seconds, then exhale, lower your arms and relax. Alternate the exercise with throwing forward different arms.

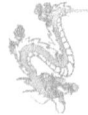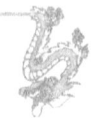

In contrast to the previous exercises, in the following exercises inhale with your nose for 4 seconds, then tense your body muscles and hold your breath for 4 seconds, relax your muscles and exhale slowly with your mouth for 4 seconds, then return to the starting position.

10. Torso slightly bent forward, arms stretched forward, palms locked together. Take a breath and at this time spread your arms apart at shoulder level and then down behind your back, bend your torso backwards. Hold your breath and maximally tense in this pose. Then exhale and relax.

11. Lean forward and touch the floor with your fingers. Inhale and straighten your body, while raising your arms in front of you and upwards, and bend your torso backwards. Tense your muscles and hold your breath. As you exhale, relax and return to the starting position.

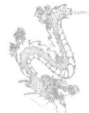
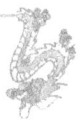

12. Stand straight. Inhale and turn your torso to the right to see the wall behind you. Stop, tense up and hold your breath. Exhale, relax and return to the starting position. Alternate rotating your torso in different directions.

13. Lie on your back, legs together, palms folded behind the back of the head, body relaxed. Breathe in through your nose for 4 seconds and lift your legs up. Tense up, hold your breath for 4 seconds and make 2 clockwise circular movements with your legs. Relax, exhale with your mouth for 4 seconds and lower your legs.

There are many different methods of absorbing energy from the outside, but the main rule is always to mentally visualize the process. To be successful, it is very important to develop an imagination of the process taking place. Do not put effort into the work of the will, as it will do little good.

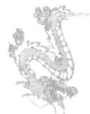
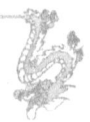

At the initial stage
of the exercises do not seek to get a lot of energy at once, as this can have a negative effect on the psyche. Do the following exercises 2 times a day for 10 minutes, preferably after waking up and before going to bed.

14. Lying on your back relax and close your eyes. When inhaling, feel the flow of pure energy, and when exhaling, direct it to the solar plexus, legs and palms. Figuratively, the flow of energy can be visualized, for example, in the form of a river or smoke. Feel how the energy moves through the body and gets to each point of the body.

15. Inhale clean energy, and on the exhalation conduct bad energy out of the body. The mental picture should be clear. Remember that not only proper breathing, but also the power of thought plays a big role in the recruitment of energy.

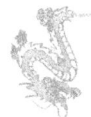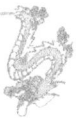

People are constantly exchanging energy between themselves and space, but there are people absorbing too much energy from others. They are called energy vampires, in their company quickly becomes uncomfortable and tiring. The absorption of energy goes through eye contact or during conversation. If you can not leave the society of these people, then store energy rhythmic breathing, close your hands and cross your legs, closing the energy flow to yourself. If another person has a very weak biofield, pay attention to this fact, it may be one of the main causes of the problem.

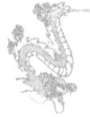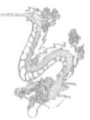

Determining
the shape of the biofield

Do the exercises 3 times a day for 10 minutes. Go to each new exercise after mastering the previous one. It is necessary to develop the ability to feel the elasticity of the biofield between the palms of your hands without any aids, such as a pendulum or a vine. Remove all jewelry from your hands and wash them well. Warm the palms of your hands by rubbing them together and they should become slightly moist. Concentrate more on the index, middle and ring fingers - these are the most sensitive elements of the hands. Relax in a standing position. Eyes closed, shoulders down, forearms bent, palms closed at the level of the lower chest, fingers slightly apart.

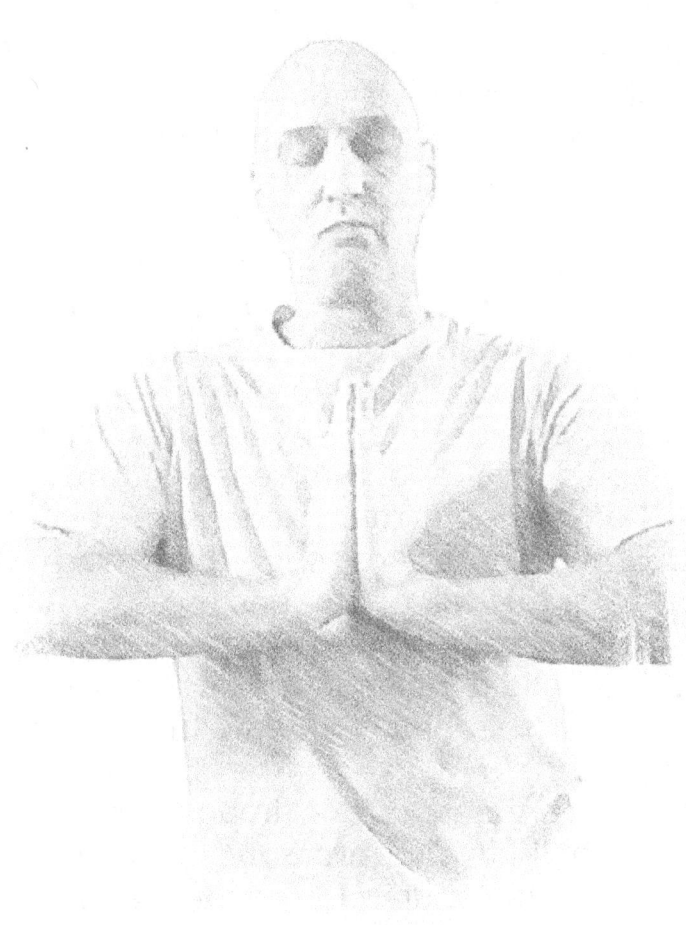

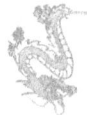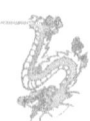

1. Inhale with your nose for 4 seconds, simultaneously move your palms away from each other and tense your arm muscles until they shake. Imagine a rubber ball glued to your palms, stretching with great effort as it increases in shape and as pure energy from space is drawn into it. Stop movement of palms on width of an elbow or a little wider, relax, hold breath for 4 seconds and make light tapping with palms on an imaginary ball, trying to feel it. When divorcing your palms, you should make one sweeping movement, and when bringing them together - two short ones. The palms are separated from each other at a distance of sensitivity, and then brought together again. There should be a feeling of slight tension of the palms when pressing on this ball. Exhale with your mouth for 4 seconds, squeeze the ball until your palms close together and imagine the energy from the ball flowing into your body. Hold your breath for 4 seconds and repeat the exercise.

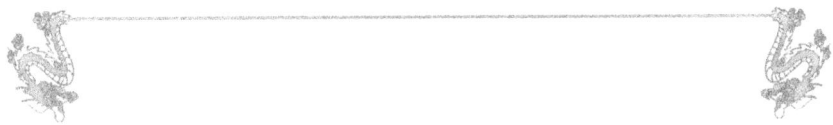

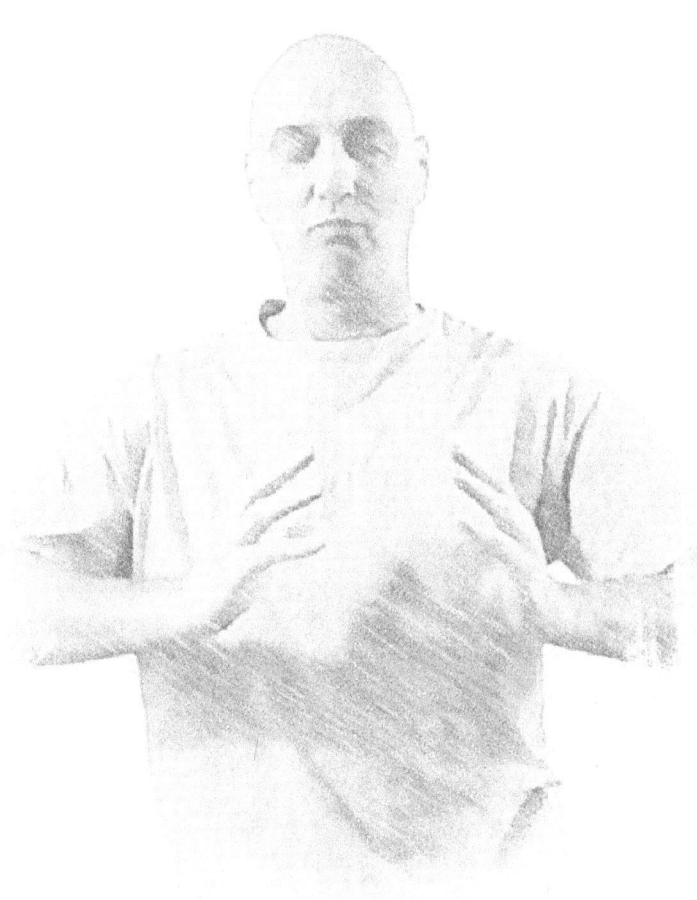

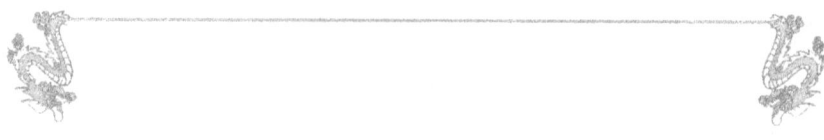

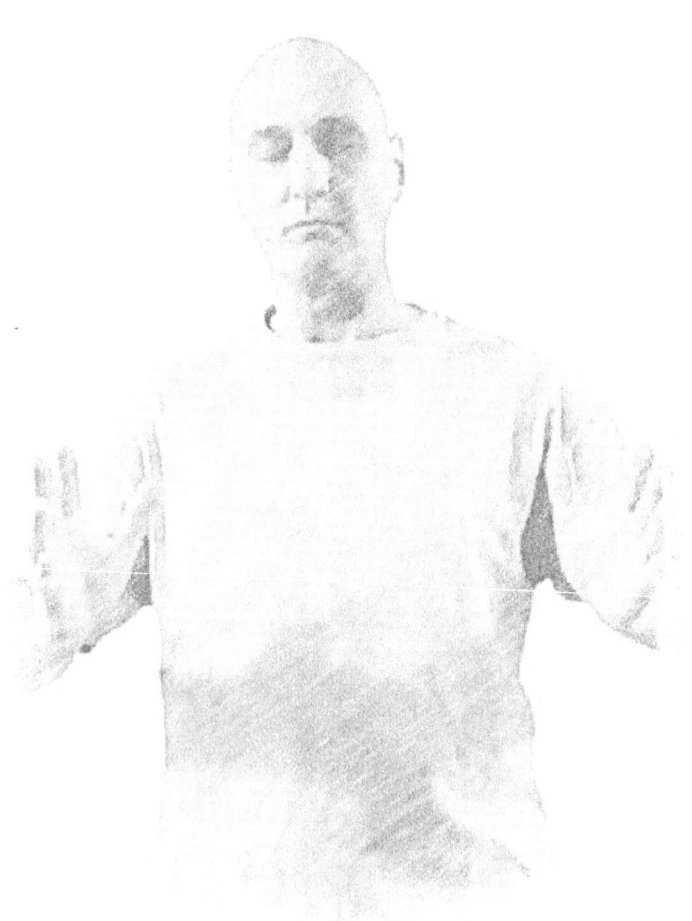

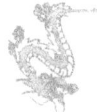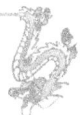

2. Try to keep as long as possible the feeling of elasticity of the biofield and not to lose the connection between the hands. Do not return each time to the initial position as in the previous exercise. Hold an energy ball in front of you, pat it lightly from different sides and feel its elasticity. Rotate it to the left and right, raise it above your head and lower it down, turn in different directions. The time cycle of rhythmic breathing is determined individually, depending on your breathing skills. However, the biofield is felt more effectively during the breath delay, so inhalation and exhalation at the first stage of training should be shorter. Having learned to feel the biofield compaction well, you can exercise with open eyes.

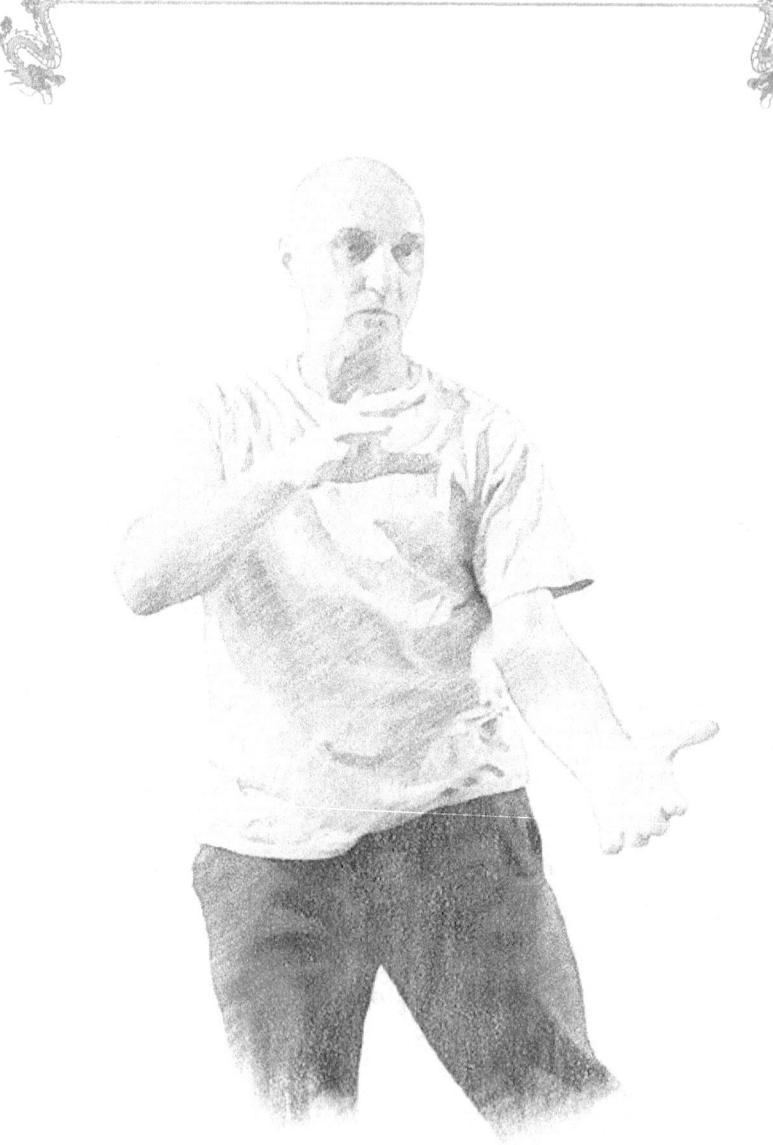

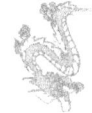
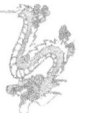
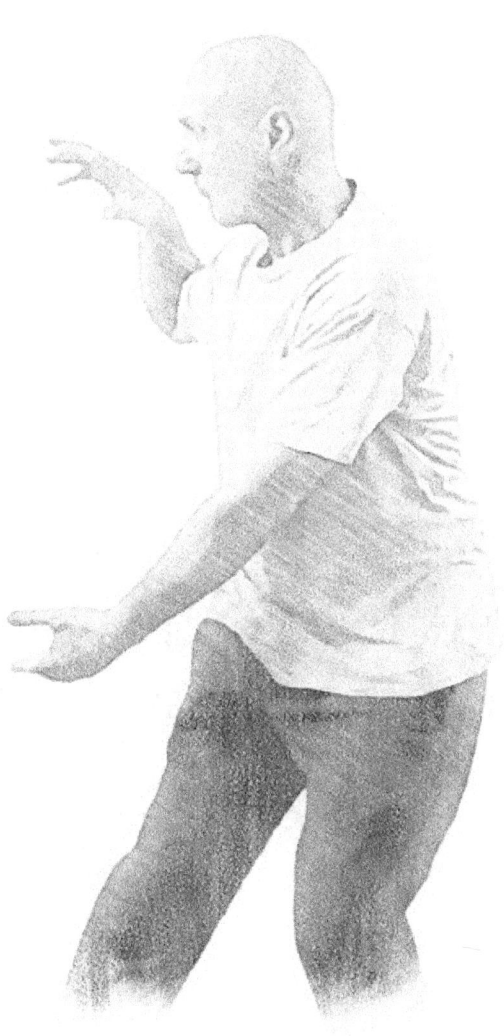

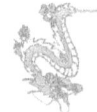
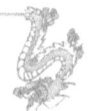

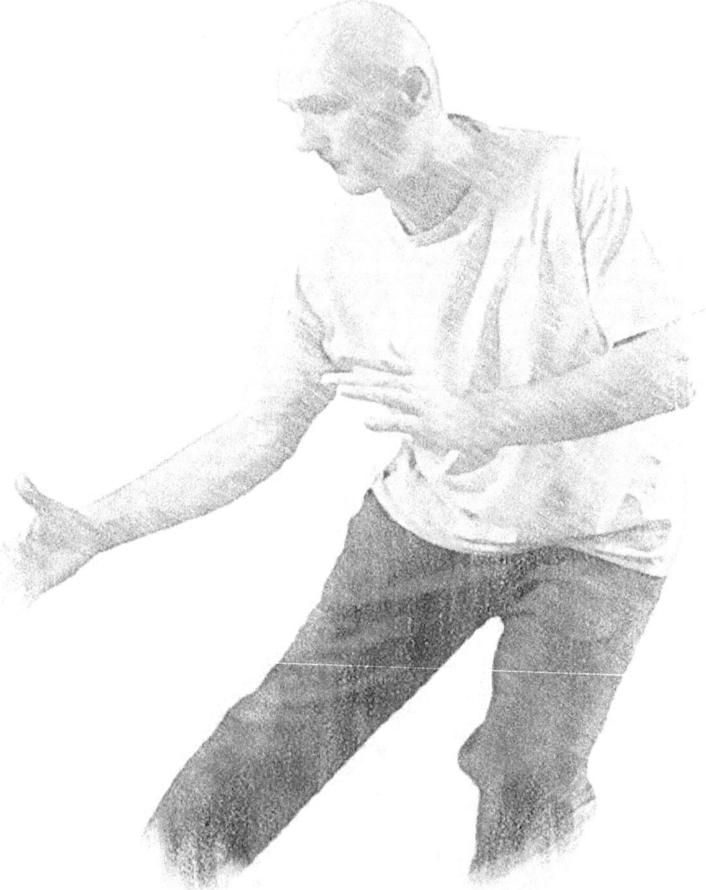

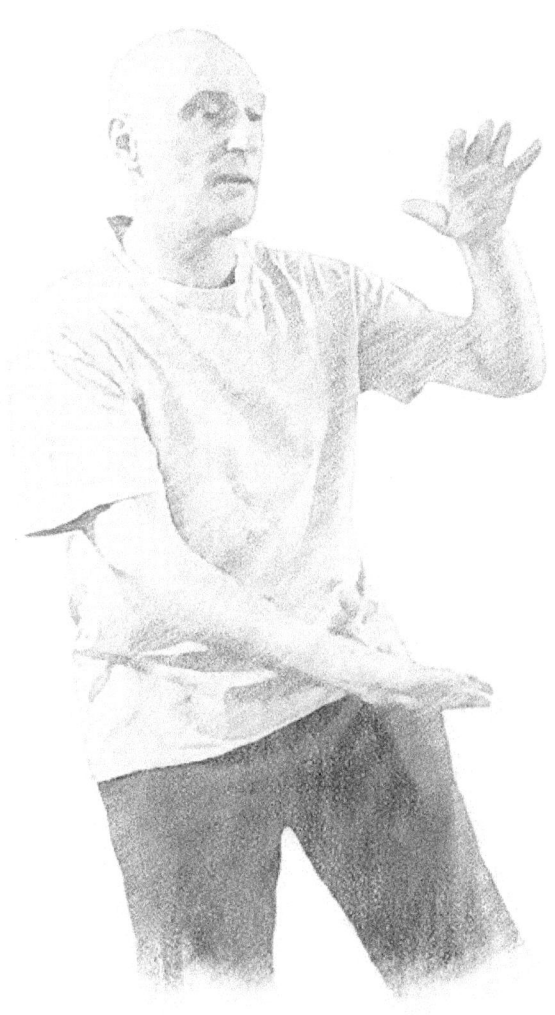

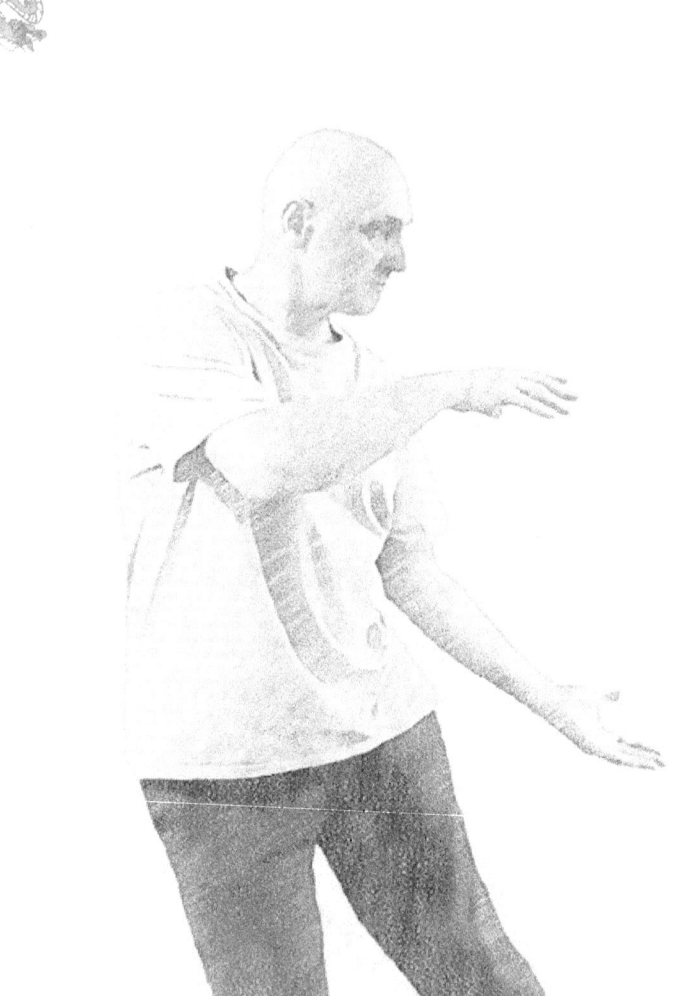

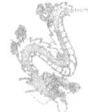
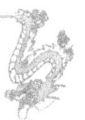
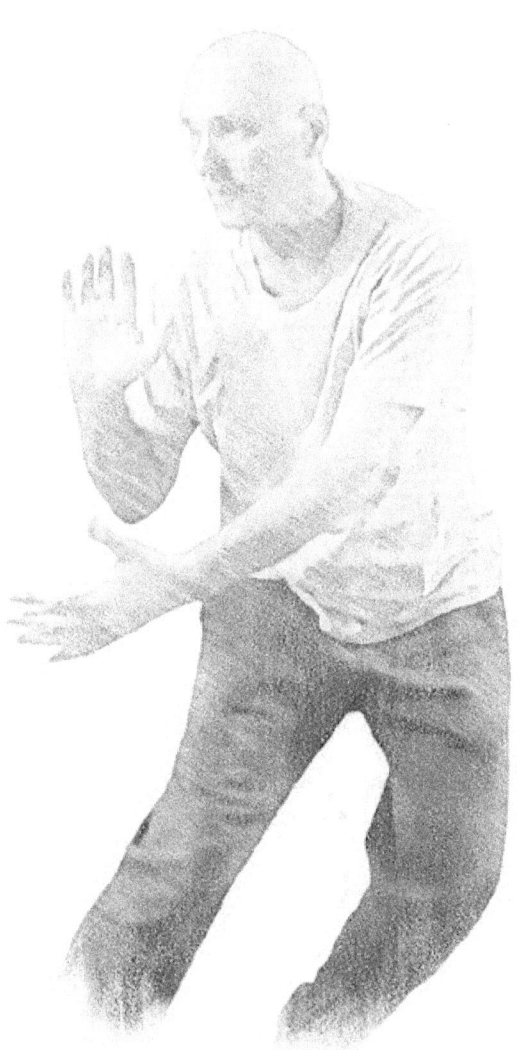

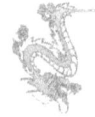
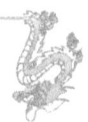

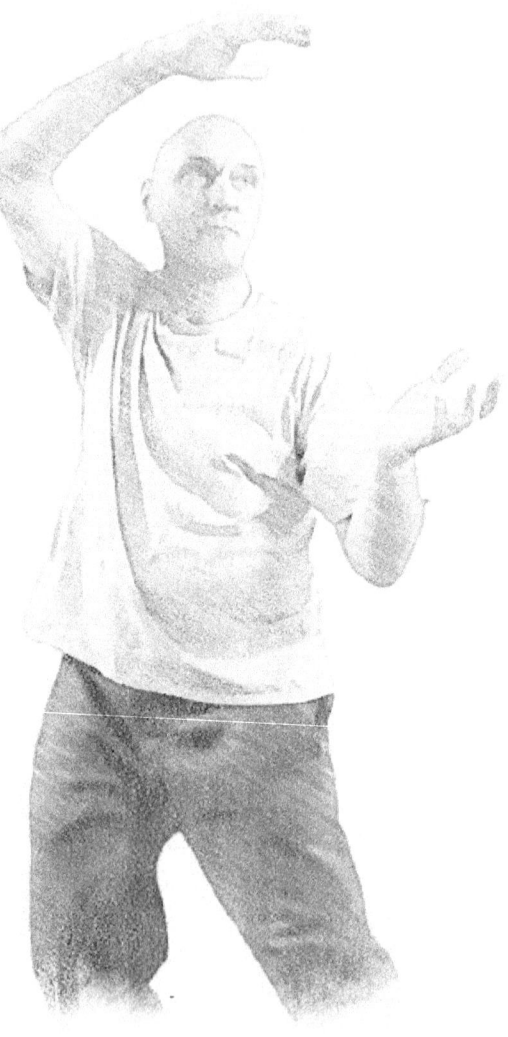

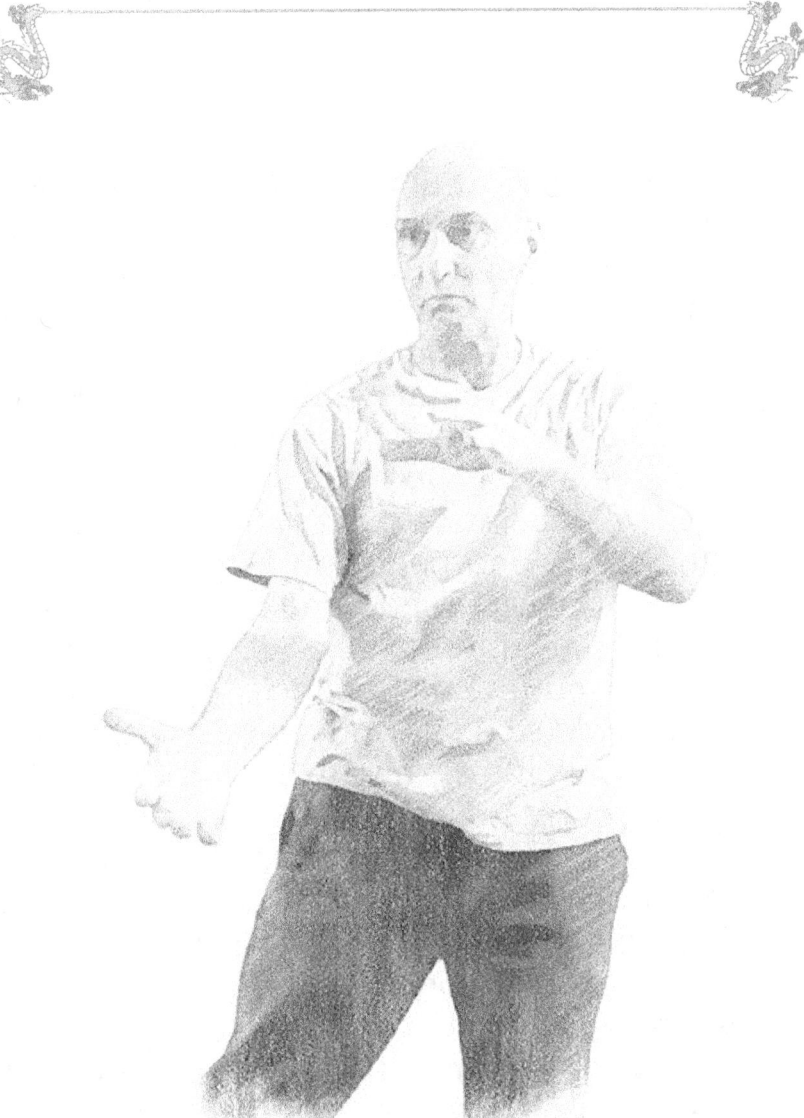

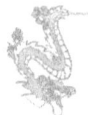
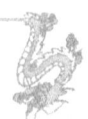

3. Establish psychological contact with a sitting or standing patient - to do this, talk about his well-being, tell him about your help and the expected result. Distracting topics of conversation can include the weather, the economy or current events. Then ask the patient to close his eyes, lower his arms along his body, relax, and be quiet. Place his chest between your palms a cubit's distance on each side and make energetic contact. Spread your palms a little wider and make several short oscillating movements back to the patient's body, until you feel the elasticity of his biofield with your palms. Raise your hands to the head area and begin a slow examination of the energy cocoon. Slowly lower your hands, slide your palms over the biofield and determine its shape and size. Finish the movement of your hands at the groin level, then with a soft quick movement raise your hands up again and repeat the cycle. If it is difficult to feel the biofield with two hands, do it first with the most sensitive hand, and use the other hand as a screen.

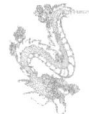
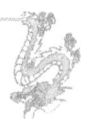

4. Feeling of the biofield from a photograph is possible by establishing an energetic contact with the patient, by analogy with a mother who subconsciously feels the pain of her child at a distance. The principle of contact is the same, only the second one is stronger. First, carefully study the photo and memorize all the features, then close your eyes and imagine this person in front of you. Then open your eyes again and compare with the original in the photo. After a stable picture in memory, close your eyes and place the imaginary patient between your palms as if at this moment a real person was being diagnosed and examine his biofield. Absence of contact can speak about death of this person.

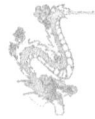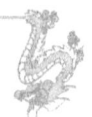

Biofield correction

Each organ has its own peak of highest activity, during which it is more amenable to treatment. In most cases, a healer corrects an area of the biofield in which there are many organs that have different peaks of activity. Therefore, we will not study the topic of biorhythms. Establish psychological contact with the patient, place him/her between your palms at a distance of a cubit on each side and even out the irregularities of his/her biofield, which have the form of hollows and hills. Keep palms parallel to each other while smoothing, squeezing and pulling out the biofield. When moving the biofield up and down, place the palms on a plane perpendicular to the body and turn them in the direction of movement. Periodically check the quality of work. Ideally, you should create the shape of an even egg from the biofield, this is the algorithm of treatment.

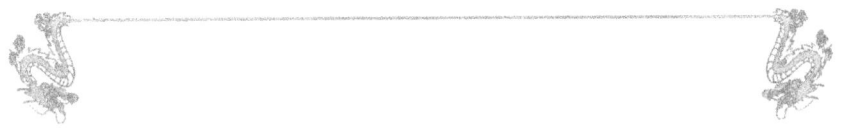

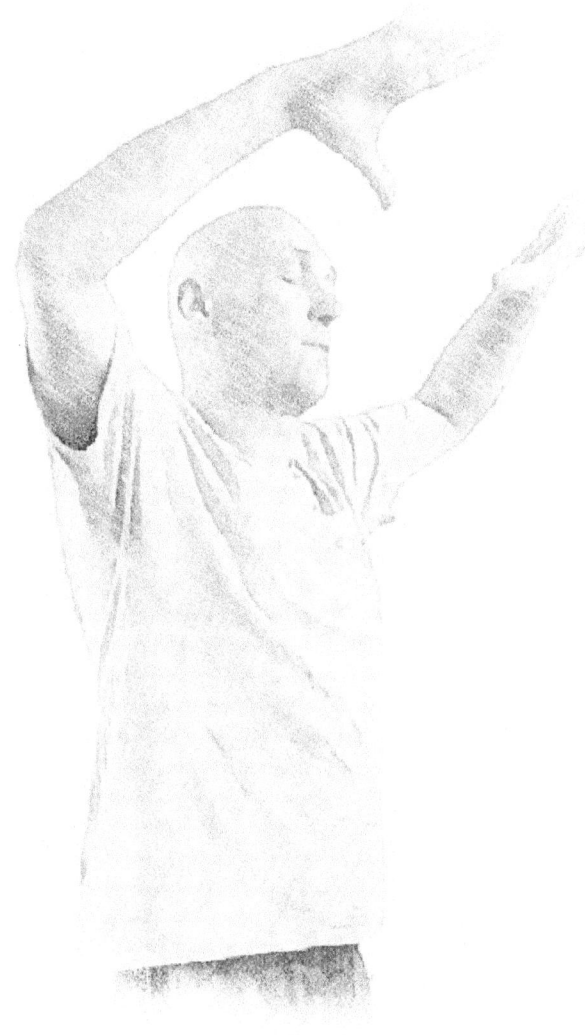

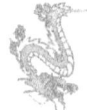
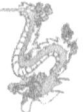

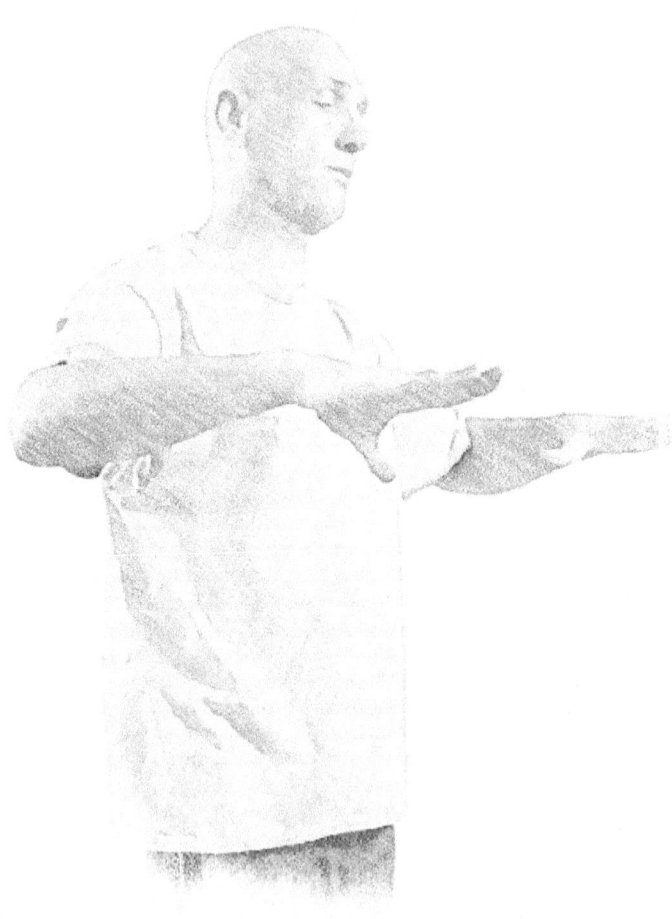

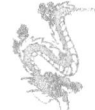
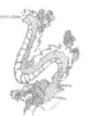
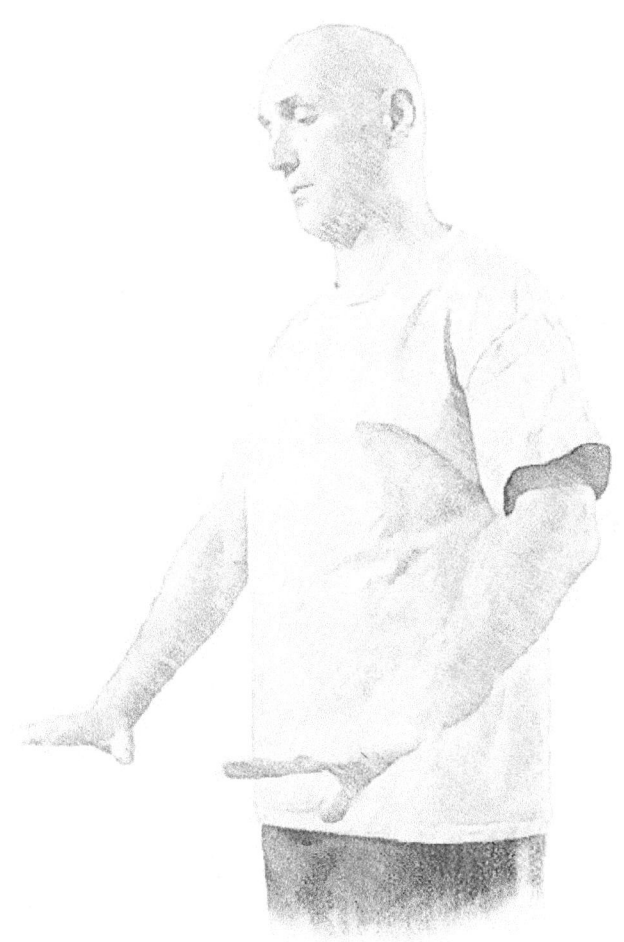

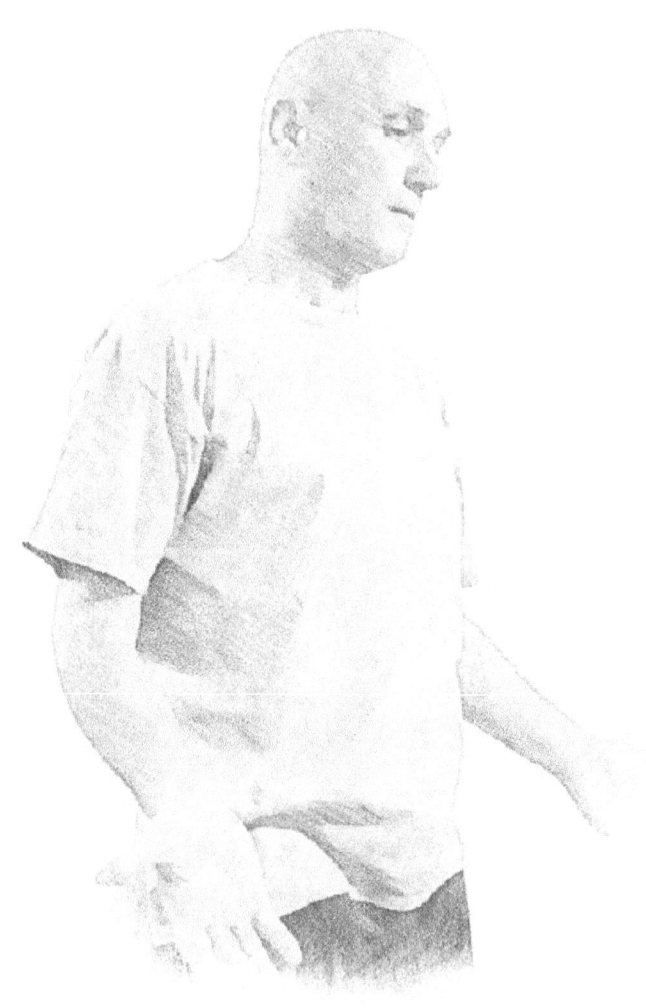

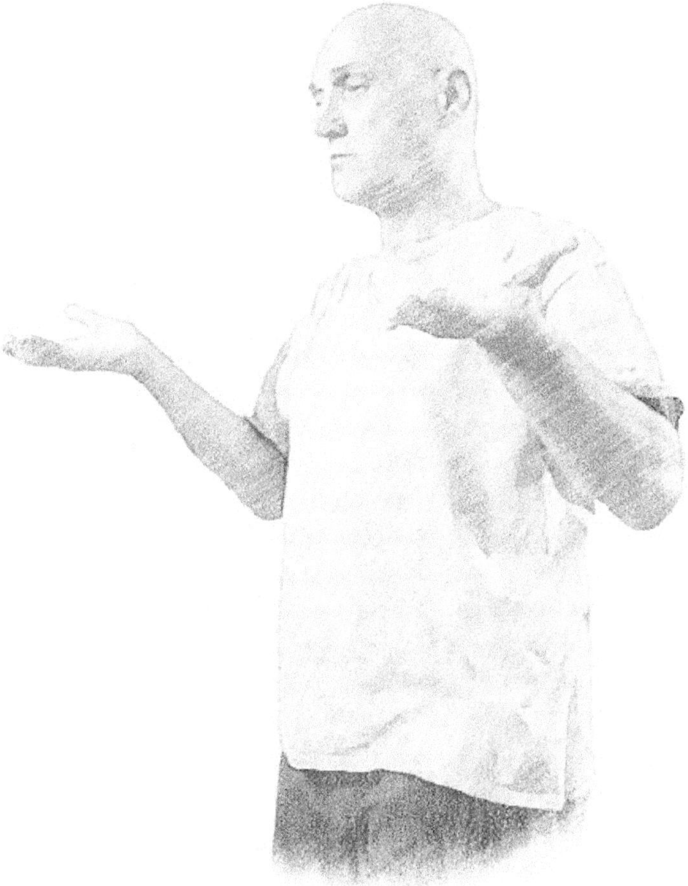

Biofield correction

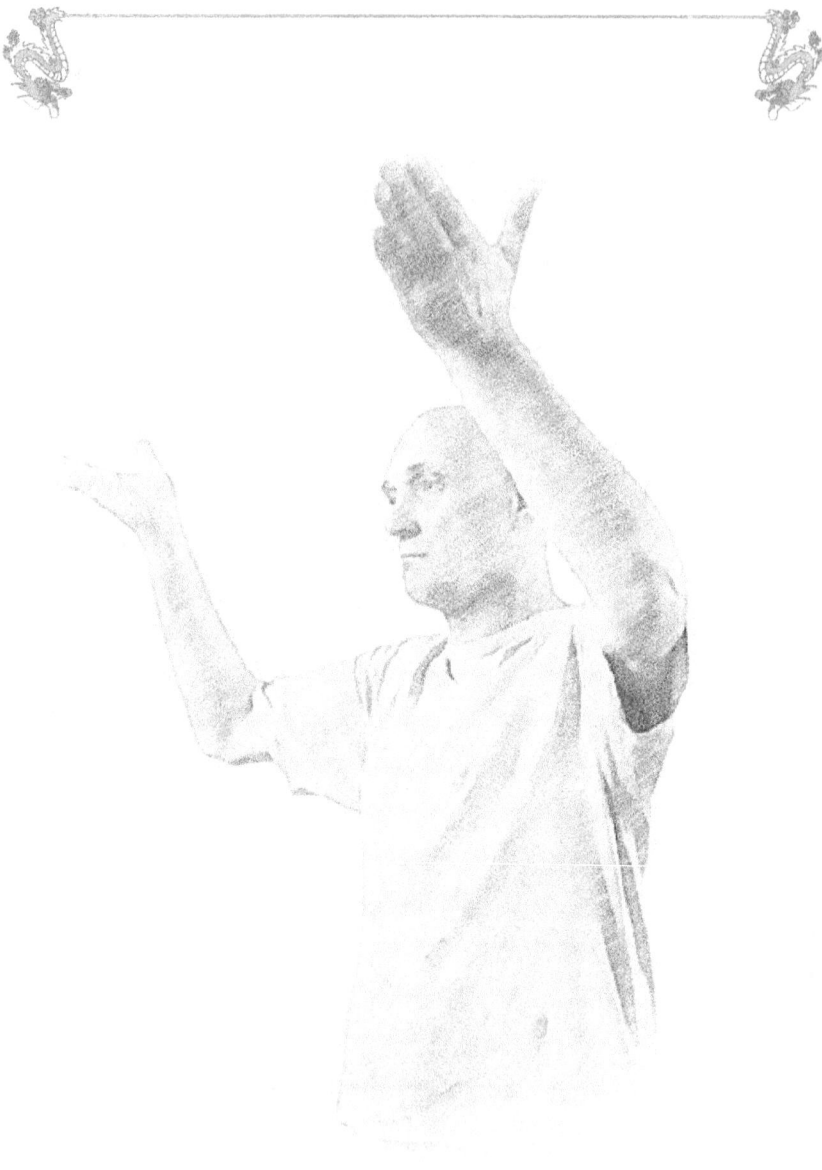

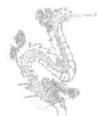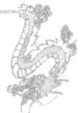

Unfortunately, it is not always possible to cure the patient at one time. Repeat the sessions again after the appearance of a pain signal, until complete stabilization. With hypertension, the hands move from above to the pelvic area, and with hypotension - vice versa. Always know the limit of your actions, because if you remove too much biofield from the head area in hypertension, the person will lose consciousness. On the contrary, if at hypotension to put a lot of energy at the top, it will lead to dizziness. Correction of the biofield should be carried out not more than half an hour a day, after which you should be sure to wash your hands.

Let's consider some practical examples.

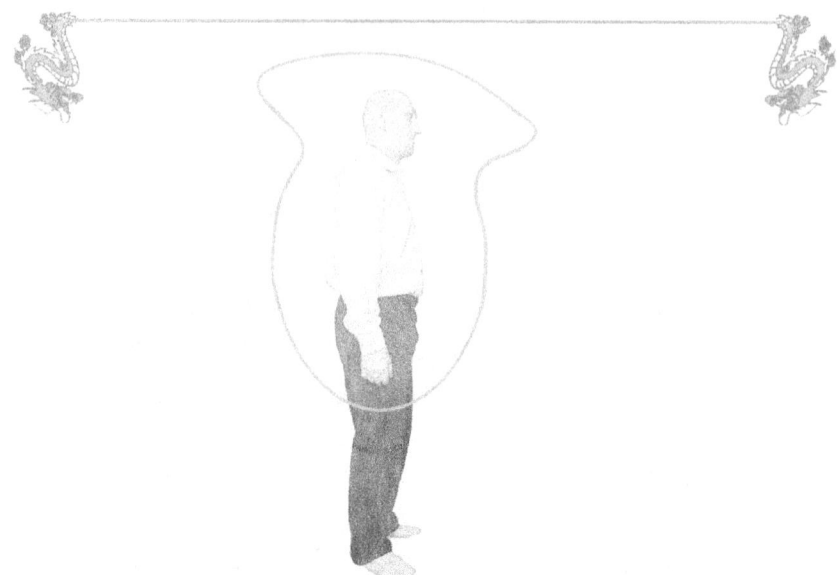

1. The patient has headaches, high blood pressure. The size of the biofield is normal, but hills are felt at the level of the cervical spine on both sides. The cause of their formation is osteochondrosis of the cervical vertebrae. It prevents the free flow of energy along the spine and spreads it to the sides like a cork. Move the excess biofield from the head to the pelvic area, the patient's condition will improve. Encourage him to visit a chiropractor, after the cause of the disease is eliminated, make a final correction of the biofield. If the plug is at the level of the chest, tracheitis and bronchitis may develop.

57

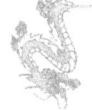
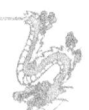
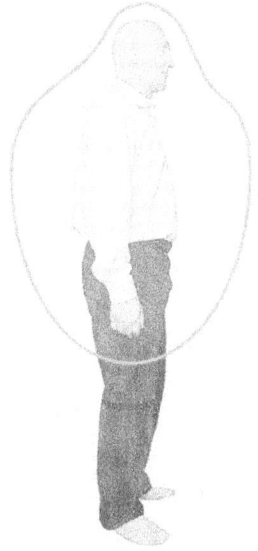

2. The patient has depression, chronic fatigue, malaise and low blood pressure. The biofield size is normal, but at the head level there are depressions on both sides and the biofield size there is a quarter of an elbow. Increase and equalize the biofield by using the lower areas as a donor.

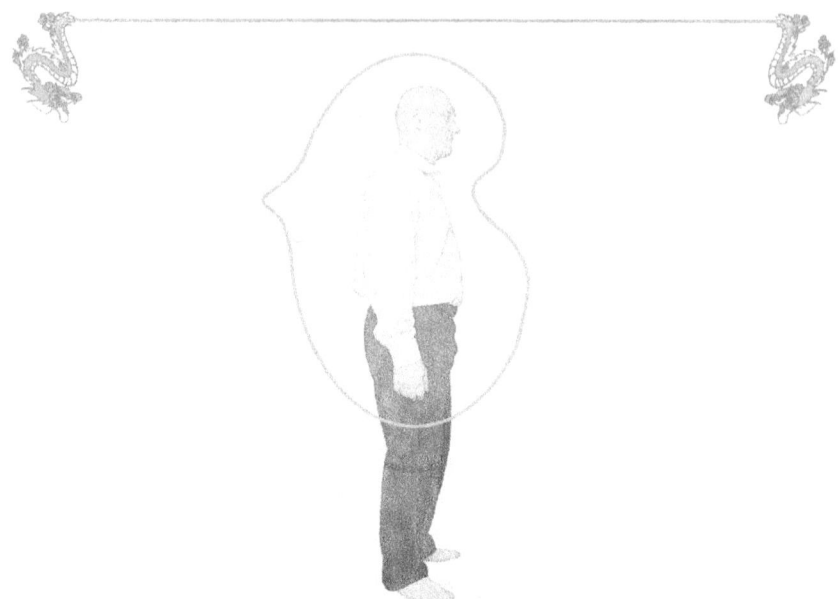

3. The patient has a sudden onset of diabetes. The size of the biofield is normal, but there are relief changes: on the chest side there is a depression and on the back side there is a hill. With the more active palm press on the hill and move towards the hollow, and with the opposite palm pull this hollow. As a rule, the disease goes away, but this combination of biofield relief is often a persistent deformation. Such deformation in the heart area can lead to a repeated heart attack if periodic biofield correction is not performed.

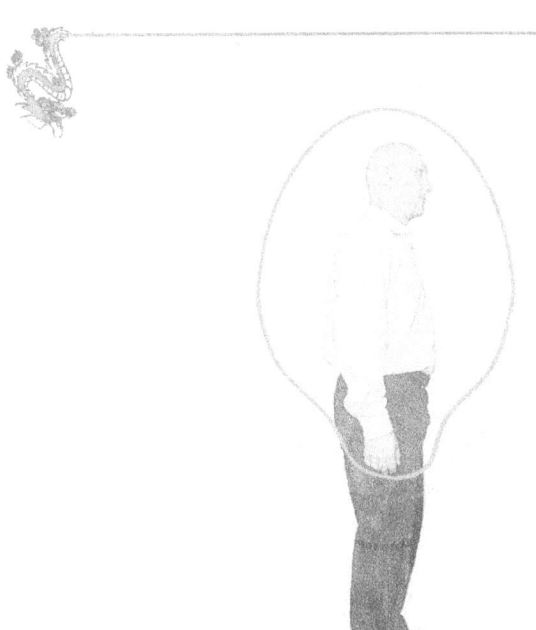

4. The patient has leukemia. The size of the biofield is normal, but in the coccyx area there are hollows on both sides. It is necessary to equalize the biofield by compensating it with the biofield from above. Usually, the symptoms of the disease will go away and the blood formula will improve. However, it is not possible to get rid of the disease completely. Correction of the biofield should be carried out periodically, because at a big break a relapse starts.

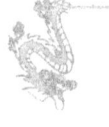
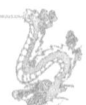
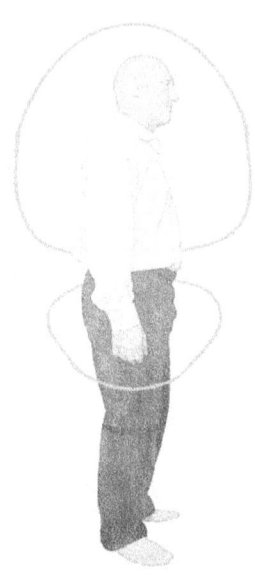

5. The patient has increased fatigue, weakness, nausea, drowsiness and enlarged lymph nodes. The size of the biofield is normal, but in the area of the navel are felt depressions on both sides, which have no bottom. At the same time the palms of the hands feel a vacuum and are pulled inside the hollow. It is almost impossible to fill this hole with biofield from other donor parts. It is likely that an early stage of cancer has been detected and a consultation with an oncologist doctor is necessary.

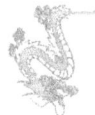
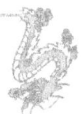

6. The patient has many different diseases and poor health. The size of the biofield is very small, only half an elbow. Its relief is uneven. In this case, you need to stimulate the whole body. Place your hands at the level of the solar plexus, with the active hand in front. After establishing energetic contact remove the shielding hand and exhale pure energy into the patient's body through the active hand. Mentally clearly visualize it coming out of the palm and flowing into the patient. Then with the middle finger of the shielding hand slowly run it upwards along the spine. Repeat the cycles and then make a diagnosis of the new biofield. The duration of this treatment is no more than 10 minutes.

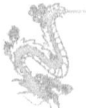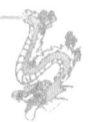

7. A patient can be treated from his/her photo if there is good energetic contact with him/her. Manipulations with hands are carried out exactly the same as when working with a real patient.

8. In self-treatment, a large set of energy automatically helps the body to heal. However, for various reasons it is not always evenly distributed throughout the body, the biofield has an uneven appearance and diseases do not go away at once. The reasons may be old diseases, vascular system disorders and so on. It is inconvenient to treat yourself, but it is necessary. Therefore, be patient and firmly know about your future victory over the disease. In a lying position put your hands on the diseased organ, inhale deeply with your nose and draw energy into your chest, then slowly exhale with your mouth and direct it exactly to the diseased organ. With the next exhalation, visualize the bad energy leaving the diseased organ. Repeat the cycles with alternating energy flows for 10 minutes 5 times a day.

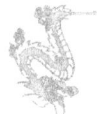 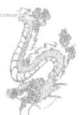

The main causes of hollows and hills in the human biofield are not only improper nutrition, various traumas, new and old diseases, but also spoilage. Anger and envy of a person gives birth to strong energetic vibrations, which can break through the biofield of the victim. Always be kind to the people around you.

Always help people in case of need, be pure of heart and unselfish.

Contents